I DO NOT SMOKE! MY HEAD IS FREE OF NICOTINE!

HOW TO BECOME A SMOKE-FREE PERSON
STEP BY STEP

1st edition

Copyright © 2020 - Markus K. Hoffmann

This book is for my family, who actively support me in all situations of life.

Content

Foreword..7

How non-smokers even get the idea to smoke 10

The dream world of tobacco advertising........ 10
Indirect advertising by smoking actors and
musicians 13
Smoking role models in everyday life 15
Why the motivation for smoking does not
disappear despite the first cigarette............... 16

**Everything revolves around nicotine when
smoking.. 18**

Direct effects of nicotine when smoking 18
Physical and psychological nicotine addiction 20
Physical addiction to nicotine 21
Nicotine tolerance 21
Physical withdrawal symptoms....................... 22
Psychological nicotine addiction..................... 23
Addiction memory and subconscious mind.... 23
Psychological withdrawal symptoms.............. 25
Nicotine addiction and health damage caused
by tobacco smoke 26

**Systematic preparation as a basis for a lasting
non-smoking life 37**

Planning the first smoke-free day.................... 38
Self-analysis as a smoker 39

Self-observation and analysis of your current smoking habits 41

Get misconceptions about smoking out of your head! 45

Anchoring the advantages of not smoking in the mind 51

Inform my environment................................. 57

Smoking the very last cigarette 58

Finally, create a smoke-free environment...... 60

Success strategies from the first day as a non-smoker 61

Successfully to the durable non-smoker in 24 - hours - steps.. 61

Avoid dicey places and situations from the outset 63

Introducing new non-smoking habits and getting rid of old smoking habits 65

Nutrient-rich food instead of tobacco smoke. 66

Addiction attacks and what you can do about them 70

Keep a written record of your non-smoking life 74

Set up a non-smoker account 75

Preventing a shift in addiction 75

How to master existential crises without relapse... 78

Hands off all nicotine products!..................... 79

Watch out! Arrogance comes before the
nicotine relapse! 84

Concluding remarks 86

Appendix 88

Foreword

Dear Readers,

I am pleased that I can help you with this book to get rid of cigarettes! As a non-smoker, you will be rewarded health-wise, financially, and generally with a better life quality!

Regardless of how many cigarettes you currently smoke every day, the path to becoming a non-smoker is always the same: You have to systematically break all of your smoking habits until everyday life without cigarettes has become entirely normal.

A preparation phase helps a successful and permanent smoking cessation, especially an analysis of your previous smoking behavior as precisely as possible. The better you know what triggers your smoking habits, the easier it is to prevent potential relapse situations.

In principle, smoking is all about the drug nicotine; the cigarette is just the packaging. In this guide, I will therefore show you the mechanisms and effects of nicotine on both your body and your psyche and how you can get rid of it.

However, this takes time because you have to switch off your addiction memory in your head in the long term. You have to relearn and consolidate your life as a non-smoker over the next few days and weeks. You have to create a new non-smoker memory in your head, on which you can then build your daily freedom from smoking.

I didn't just become a non-smoker from one moment to the next. At that time, I was still an avid smoker and couldn't imagine a day without cigarettes. It went so far that my friends and I went to a smokers' cinema several times, where we "indulged" our nicotine addiction.

But then my enthusiasm for smoking waned a lot when I began to have bleeding gums and holey teeth. At the time, my dentist warned me urgently against continued smoking with the words: »You have to stop smoking!« In addition to my dental problems, there were also recurring laryngitis and infections.

I decided to quit smoking, but initially, I used the wrong method: I just wanted to smoke less and become completely smoke-free. But unfortunately, that didn't work in the long term; I fell back on my old cigarette quota.

After this setback, I began to do intensive research on smoking. I also tried different smoking cessation programs. My image of smoking as a hobby and a relaxed lifestyle increasingly collapsed.

I systematically prepared my quit smoking and then finally managed to get rid of the cigarettes. This book has summarized exactly those strategies that have helped me and numerous other ex-smokers succeed for years. I am convinced that these experiences and knowledge will also help you to lead a free and self-determined life again finally!

I now wish you the best of luck and success with this guide, and I would be delighted if you soon belong to the group of happy non-smokers!

Markus K. Hoffmann

How non-smokers even get the idea to smoke

What was your motivation to take up a cigarette? Was it the idea of adventure, freedom, coolness, community spirit, or relaxation? As a non-smoker, what rewards did you hope to get from smoking?

In any case, like all the other 1.1 billion smokers in the world, you did not have the desire to become a smoker from birth. You were tempted by various external influences to reach for a cigarette. Even as a child, you were sometimes confronted with cigarette advertisements, smoking people in movies and television, or by other smoking role models in everyday life. They told you:

"SMOKING MAKES LIFE BETTER, START SMOKING TOO! «

The dream world of tobacco advertising

Which images do you spontaneously associate with cigarette advertisements? Do you think of emaciated, cancer-stricken chain smokers who light a cigarette with pleasure? People with a smoker's leg? Or smokers in general who smile into the camera with rotten teeth and oral cavity cancer?

Of course not! Smokers in tobacco advertising are young, slim, and healthy-looking people. Women are thin, successful, and emancipated women with flawless complexion.

Mostly teenagers and young adults are important customers for the tobacco industry. They are not yet so concerned about the health consequences and are easily attracted to smoking's so-called adventure. They are crucial for a cigarette brand to expand with new customers. Tobacco advertising pulls out all the stops to combine cigarettes with youthfulness, sexual attractiveness, and adventure. This strategy is particularly objectionable because the earlier young people start smoking, the more harmful it is for them in the long term.

I came into contact with cigarette advertisements in the cinema when I was still a young adult. For example, I can remember a commercial with a stunt pilot who, after some daredevil maneuvers, lit a cigarette with relish. At first glance, this commercial was impressive, and to a certain extent, it certainly encouraged me to continue smoking. In retrospect, I can only shake my head over it.

A few decades ago, cigarettes were still advertised in motorsports, especially in Formula 1. Entire racing cars were plastered with cigarette advertising. In this context, smoking stood for sporting performance, daredevilry, and heroism. In the seventies, there were even racing drivers who smoked themselves. Fortunately, a complete ban on advertising has become established in this area.

Logically, the tobacco industry aims to attract new customers and keep existing customers at the (cigarette) pole. It is always thinking up new product variants to bind customers to their preferred brand in the long term. By introducing so-called light cigarettes or special editions, health-conscious smokers are calmed down so that they can continue smoking in peace. The design of the pack is also essential. It communicates directly with the smoker and becomes his status symbol, which accompanies him everywhere.

Overall, a tobacco advertising ban is particularly crucial to reduce the number of smokers. As a comprehensive study[1] by the US National Cancer Institute shows, advertising in the media influences especially young people in their smoking behavior. Under the influence of tobacco advertising, this target group tends to reach for a cigarette and smoke habitually later on.

In the countries of the European Union, the ban on tobacco advertising is now firmly established. For example, in most member countries, billboard advertising in public places and tobacco advertising in newspapers and on the Internet is prohibited.

However, tobacco advertising takes place worldwide indirectly in social media, especially YouTube. Influencers, more or less, openly advertise smoking in their lifestyle videos. Meanwhile, however, Instagram, for example, has announced that it will block users who promote e-cigarettes, tobacco products, and weapons. Other companies will hopefully follow this positive example in the future.

Indirect advertising by smoking actors and musicians

Especially in the early cinema phase with acting greats like Humphrey Bogart or Marlene Dietrich, smoking was very present. Bogart often played a regular chain smoker, who embodied the hardened, cool hero and gave smoking an attractive image with his striking face and gestures.

Marlene Dietrich, in turn, conveyed to the audience the image of the emancipated, strong woman and combined smoking with glamour and world fame. All this she embodied at the same time as a singer.

The epitome of the smoking rebel was James Dean in the 50s. While smoking, he rebelled against the conventions of the 1950s and "inspired" a whole generation of young people worldwide.

Especially in the Westerns of the following decades, smoking cowboys were to be seen repeatedly, of course, first and foremost, John Wayne. The Marlboro Man's connection is so evident that one can almost no longer speak of indirect advertising.

Of course, the then still smoking James Bond alias Sean Connery also stands out, the epitome of the smart, well-trained agent in whom all women become "weak." This screen hero conveys to the viewer that cigarette smoking is easily compatible with physical health and fitness. Moreover, his obligatory drink became the status symbol of the agent. Here, alcohol and cigarettes were genuinely mystified.

While smoking remained present on the silver screen in the 70s and 80s, the protection of non-smokers became increasingly important in the following decades. Smoking was increasingly frowned upon in the western industrial nations, and the smoking heroes and heroines increasingly disappeared from the movies. However, a trend reversal is taking place in recent times. In cult series and films such as "Orange is the new Black" or "Once Upon a Time in Hollywood," smoking protagonists can be seen time and again. Once Upon a Time in Hollywood," also conjures up a golden era in which everyone still had the "freedom" to smoke. This development is very negative overall. Hopefully, there will be a rethink within the film industry, or people, in general, will retake a stand against smoking.

Smoking role models in everyday life

Smoking role models in everyday life are incredibly crucial for non-smokers to reach for a cigarette themselves. Parents certainly have the most substantial influence on their children.

A study by [2]European researchers published in 2010 in the Oxford Bulletin of Economics and Statistics shows that children of smokers are much more likely to reach for cigarettes later than non-smokers. Above all, this applies in a gender-specific way between father and son or mother and daughter.

By the parents' automatic role model function, smoking is anchored in the child's head as usual and acceptable. Therefore, by stopping smoking, you can save yourself and your children a lot of harm.

The circle of friends is the second major factor for starting to smoke. Especially parties with friends and visits to smoking establishments can be the trigger. Significantly if enormous quantities of alcohol flow, the danger rises to seize the cigarette because nicotine and alcohol rock each other highly in their effect on the brain.

Especially at the beginning of your non-smoking life, it will be essential to avoid the situations mentioned above as much as possible. The most important motto is:

Why the motivation for smoking does not disappear despite the first cigarette

Do you still remember how you had your first cigarette? Were you persuaded spontaneously, or did you toy with the idea long before? Were you nervous or merely full of anticipation? Did you secretly smoke alone in a hiding place or together with your smoking friends?

I still remember my first cigarette well. My friends and I were sitting together at home while everyone was smoking but me. Suddenly I felt the urge to join in. I joyfully took my very first cigarette in my hand and clumsily lit it.

And with the first pulmonary pull, I experienced what, in principle, happens to every smoker in the beginning: I coughed and had the feeling of not breathing. I got dizzy and sick. I heard my friends in the background, making fun of my pale complexion.

In any case, at the very beginning of my smoking career, my body had issued an unmistakable warning:

LET'S GET OUT WITH THE POISONOUS STUFF!

This reaction of the body is entirely logical. Since tobacco smoke virtually robs the smoker of the air he breathes and carbon monoxide sabotages the absorption of oxygen in the blood, the body now sets off all the alarm bells!

In retrospect, the following question now arises: Why do smokers continue after this negative experience? How does tobacco smoke suddenly become bearable or even pleasure?

At this point, the previously mentioned factors come into play: the cigarette's positive image and the smoking role models. Besides, there is the typical "smoker's advice" that you have undoubtedly heard from other smokers: "It's quite normal at the beginning, you get used to it soon! It goes away soon! It was the same with us; that is quite normal!" All of this is not the smoker's fault. They are themselves victims of tobacco propaganda and the tobacco machine!

The new smoker will not give up after the first cigarette. He tells himself absurd things like: "I just have to get used to it, everybody does! So he continues to smoke. Soon he comes to the point where he is addicted to cigarettes, i.e., addicted to nicotine.

We will now take a closer look at this drug in the next section.

Everything revolves around nicotine when smoking

Nicotine is a nerve poison that the tobacco plant produces against predators. The craving for this poison currently drives more than 1.1 billion smokers worldwide into an addiction to cigarettes. According to the WHO World Tobacco Report of 2019, tobacco smoke kills over 8 million people every year. Nicotine has, by far, an enormous effect when smoking tobacco compared to all other nicotine products. In less than 10 seconds, the nerve poison shoots into the smoker's brain. Because of this, you perceive the self-poisoning by cigarettes as a reward and pleasure.

Direct effects of nicotine when smoking

By burning the tobacco, the nerve poison is released and absorbed through the tobacco smoker's lungs. It is then distributed throughout the body via the bloodstream. The nicotine reaches the brain in less than 10 seconds. There it docks on specific nerve cells, the so-called nicotine receptors. The body's messenger substance acetylcholine, which influences vital body functions such as breathing, blood pressure, heartbeat, digestion, and metabolism, otherwise acts on these nerve cells. The nicotine kick in the brain stimulates these nerve cells. The body reacts by releasing messenger substances such as dopamine, adrenaline, and endorphins, giving the smoker a short-term high. The nicotine sets various physical processes in motion. The most important of these are:

- The heart rate increases.

- Blood pressure increases due to the narrowing of the blood vessels.

- The breathing frequency increases; the breath becomes shallower.

- The skin is less supplied with blood and cools down.

- Blood sugar is increasingly released.

- Stomach activity and digestion are forced.

- The stress hormone cortisol is released more strongly.

- The risk of thrombosis increases because the tendency of the blood to clot increases.

Physical and psychological nicotine addiction

The consumption of nicotine sooner or later leads to physical and psychological addiction, depending on the user's constitution. Especially on the psychological level, nicotine has a strong influence on the smoker's behavior. Nicotine works most strongly in the cigarette. That's because of the fast absorption rate of nicotine and the artificial additives added to the cigarette.

Nicotine addicts show the following behavior patterns:

- ➢ the strong psychological compulsion to consume the narcotic, the so-called craving
- ➢ loss of control over the extent of consumption
- ➢ the occurrence of a physical tolerance
- ➢ systematic neglect of everyday interests due to addiction
- ➢ the continuation of consumption despite negative physical, psychological and social effects

Do not be alarmed if you recognize your current behavior on this list. Instead, motivate yourself all the more to finally break out of this devil circle. No matter how much you have already smoked, everyone has the chance to make it.

Physical addiction to nicotine

Nicotine addiction manifests itself physically on the one hand through the withdrawal symptoms; on the other hand, it develops a body's tolerance towards nicotine. The extent of physical addiction depends on the individual smoker.

Nicotine tolerance

The constant intake of nicotine causes an increased release of dopamine in the brain, causing the natural dopamine system to lose its balance.

To bring the body's system back under control, the body's throttles the production of dopamine. Nicotine tolerance develops, i.e., the body gradually gets used to the effect of nicotine, and the smoker needs more and more nicotine to achieve the same effect as before. The number of nicotinic receptors in the brain increases steadily. The smoker is getting more and more addicted.

Physical withdrawal symptoms

Practically every smoker has already felt withdrawal symptoms in his or her smoking life. It's all about the constant up and down of the blood's nicotine level, which transports the nicotine to the brain's nicotinic receptors.

After each cigarette, the nicotine level rises briefly but drops significantly again within an hour. The more dependent the smoker is on nicotine, the sooner the first withdrawal symptoms begin, whereby the nicotinic receptors in the brain increasingly demand nicotine. With a new cigarette, the smoker is then "relieved" of stress for a short time, until the whole nasty game starts all over again. The most common withdrawal symptoms are as follows:

- tremble
- tingling
- headache
- sweats
- nausea
- constipation
- increased feeling of hunger

Overall, withdrawal symptoms depend on the individual's physical condition and how addicted the individual smoker already is. In the first phase of your withdrawal, you will mainly experience physical withdrawal symptoms. This phase usually ends within a week. You will feel

the most substantial withdrawal symptoms after 3-4 days, and then they will gradually go away. After seven days, most of the nicotinic receptors that have been additionally created by smoking will already be gone.

Psychological nicotine addiction

During and after cigarette smoking, processes take place systematically in your head that make you psychologically dependent. Every nicotine kick is stored in your brain, along with the events during smoking. If, for example, you are having a perfect time at a party and smoke while you are doing so, your brain links these two experiences and creates new nerve connections. Just like all other experiences with cigarettes, this memory becomes a part of the so-called addiction memory.

Addiction memory and subconscious mind

The addiction memory is the linchpin of nicotine addiction—it stores all memories with a "positive" reference to smoking. The nerve pathways of the addiction memory are formed in those areas of the brain based on a robust stimulus-response pattern. The driving force of the addiction memory is nicotine:

- On the one hand, it docks to the reward center of your brain.

- On the other hand, it activates the area of the brain associated with learning and long-term memory.

By repeating a cigarette smoking countless times, you automatically reach for the cigarette over time, and your smoking routines run again and again as in autopilot mode. Smoking has now dug deep into your subconscious mind.

To break down these behaviors, you have to relearn all the actions connected with the cigarette. The whole process takes time and patience, whereby you can establish your non-smoking routines for the most part in your head over 5 to 6 weeks.

The current research state suggests that while you can reduce your addiction memory to a small extent, it is impossible to erase it. Individual nerve tracts with memories of smoking will remain with you.

Therefore it can happen that ex-smokers suddenly feel like smoking even after months or even years of not smoking due to a visual stimulus. For example, when you see someone smoking your former cigarette brand or when you return to a place where you used to smoke a lot. Stay calm in these situations, and consistently continue your non-smoking path. In the book's further course, I will show you effective antidotes and how you can survive such conditions unharmed.

Psychological withdrawal symptoms

The psychological withdrawal symptoms, like the physical ones, vary in intensity from smoker to smoker. To free yourself from these withdrawal symptoms, you need patience and consistent action. I have listed the most common psychological symptoms for you here:

- Irritability

- inner restlessness

- depressed mood

- difficulty concentrating

- anxiety disorders

- the constant circling of thoughts about the addictive substance nicotine

- the so-called craving, a moment of intense desire

With the strategies you will find in the following chapters, you can get most of these psychological withdrawal symptoms under control after a few weeks.

Nicotine addiction and health damage caused by tobacco smoke

The driving force to reach for a cigarette, is, as we saw earlier, nicotine addiction. It opens the door to tobacco smoke to poison the smoker. The burning cigarette contains over 250 poisonous and over 70 proven carcinogenic substances[3]. Every time you light a cigarette, you start a radioactive and chemical attack on your body.

I have listed below a selection of the most harmful substances in the cigarette to show you which poison you are drawing in with every puff on the cigarette.

Tar

Tar is a liquid black-brown hydrocarbon mixture that forms in the smoker's lungs from tobacco smoke. It is full of carcinogenic toxins. If you smoke 20 cigarettes a day, you will empty the equivalent of one cup of tar into your lungs each year. It sticks the cilia in the airways and lungs. Dust can no longer be coughed out, and you will be poisoned step by step.

Carbon Monoxide

It is produced only if tobacco burns. Carbon Monoxide is a colorless, odorless gas. It forms during the incomplete combustion of carbonaceous objects and inhibits oxygen on the red blood cells. Thus, the body gets less oxygen, leading to a lack of concentration, nausea, and shortness of breath. In high concentrations, carbon monoxide can lead to death. Especially unborn children in the womb are at risk from carbon monoxide.

Polycyclic aromatic hydrocarbons (PAH)

They are in tobacco smoke or car exhaust fumes, among other things. PAHs are formed by the incomplete combustion of organic material such as wood, coal, or oil and cause tumors in the respiratory tract. Many PAHs have carcinogenic, mutagenic, and reprotoxic properties and accumulate throughout the body.

The leading representative is benzpyrene. In this process, the tumor suppressor gene p53 is damaged, thereby switching off a cancer growth brake in the cells.

Formaldehyde

Formaldehyde is a colorless, pungent-smelling gas. It arises in the cigarette by burning off the added sugar. Formaldehyde irritates the respiratory tract, mucous membranes can swell, and the eyes' conjunctiva is attacked. It can cause headaches, tiredness, and concentration problems and damage the central nervous system. The toxin is also associated with the development of allergies and asthmatic complaints. Formaldehyde can cause cancer of the nasopharynx in the long term.

Nitrosamines

They are poisonous, nitrogenous compounds that occur in tobacco and emerge, for example, during smoking or grilling. Nitrosamines are formed by the combination of amines with nitrite and are converted in our body into the formaldehyde described above. Nitrosamines are associated with various types of cancer and also damage the liver.

Arsenic

This element occurs in nature in different toxic variants. The smoker inhales the carcinogenic inorganic arsenic. This form of arsenic reaches all organs, and the long-term intake of this poison can cause skin damage, heart disease, and lung damage. Inorganic arsenic is also found in various rice types in varying concentrations, depending on how the rice is grown and cooked.

Hydrogen cyanide

Hydrogen cyanide is a highly toxic, colorless liquid absorbed as a gas through the lungs when smoking. Although this gas is only present in cigarettes in tiny quantities, it can cause headaches, nausea, and vomiting. Hydrogen cyanide has an effect on cellular respiration; above a specific dose, internal suffocation sets in. The Nazis used Hydrogen cyanide (the horrifying Zyklon B) in Extermination Camps during World War II.

Polonium

Polonium is a radioactive decay product of uranium. It enters the tobacco leaves via the air or from the soil via the roots. The tobacco plant stores radioactive substances particularly well. Polonium is a highly aggressive alpha emitter that radiates the smoker's lungs from within and can lead to lung cancer.

Plutonium

The well-known Plutonium is used in atomic bombs and nuclear power plants. Through satellite crashes in the sixties and seventies, Plutonium was released into the atmosphere and finally into the tobacco plant. Plutonium has a strong carcinogenic effect.

The radioactive radiation in cigarette smoke is a particularly dangerous source of DNA mutations. If you smoke two packs of cigarettes a day, this is equivalent to 250 x-rays a year!

Additives added to the cigarette by the manufacturers

The manufacturers mix today's industrially produced cigarettes with hundreds of different additives. These have a significant influence on the tobacco's effect and a decisive impact on the addictive potential, i.e., nicotine intake. (More on this in the next chapter). The tobacco companies have a wide margin of maneuver in what they can add to the cigarettes.

Cigarettes have additives for several reasons. They give the cigarette its taste, regulate the cigarette's burning speed, and keep the tobacco moist to a certain degree. Also, they partly promote nicotine addiction. These additives are supposed to make the cigarette more attractive, which also plays an essential role in e-cigarettes. More about this later.

Although some additives are foods from everyday use, they become partly carcinogenic chemical compounds in the hot cigarette embers at over 600 degrees.

Here I have listed some of these toxic compounds:

Sugar or sugar-containing substances

Sugar or sugar-containing substances such as honey, cereals, caramel, or maple syrup are added to tobacco by cigarette manufacturers for taste reasons. When the cigarette burns down, most of the sugar is chemically converted, and harmful compounds called aldehydes, for example, formaldehyde, are produced.

Menthol

In individual cigarettes, menthol capsules are embedded in the filter, making tobacco smoke more pleasant and tolerant. Besides, the advertising gives the menthol a "freshness kick." These cigarette brands are aimed primarily at young newcomers. However, menthol in no way has a health benefit; on the contrary, menthol causes the smoke to be inhaled more in-depth into the bronchi. Also, the partial combustion of menthol produces the carcinogenic substances benzpyrene and benzene.

Fortunately, since 20.5.2020, the sale of menthol cigarettes has been banned in the entire EU.

Ammonium compounds

Combustion during smoking produces ammonia from the
added ammonium compounds. It is a poisonous, pun-
gent gas. It causes the nicotine kick to be more decisive
and last longer. The lungs can absorb the nicotine faster,
and the brain is flooded with nicotine.

**Humectants such as glycerin or propanediol (also
known as propylene glycol)**

Propanediol is a colorless liquid. Burning it produces
toxic propylene oxide, which irritates the skin, eyes, and
respiratory tract.

Glycerine is used in various areas, such as food, cleaning
agents, and medicines. While smoking, acrolein emerges,
which irritates the respiratory tract. Besides, this para-
lyzes the self-cleaning apparatus in the bronchi.

The most common diseases caused by smoking

Due to all the previously mentioned toxins in the cigarette, many smokers suffer from various serious diseases:

Lung diseases - lung cancer, asthma, COPD

Tobacco smoke causes the most significant possible damage, especially in the lungs. It causes various inflammatory processes, damages the lung tissue, and promotes the formation of bronchial mucus. 9 out of 10 lung cancers are due to smoking. The risk of lung cancer increases continuously with the years of smoking and the number of cigarettes smoked. A significant increase in lung cancer in women has been observed in recent years.

Asthma, which is accompanied by chronic inflammation of the airways, can be triggered and aggravated by smoking. This applies to both active and passive smoking.

Chronic smoker's bronchitis (COPD) is also promoted by smoking. The symptoms of this disease are chronic cough, shortness of breath, and sputum. Ninety percent of all COPD patients were ex-smokers.

Regardless of how long you have been smoking, you should definitely stay in contact with a lung specialist to closely observe your lungs.

Heart disease and stroke

The heart is also massively damaged by tobacco smoke. Many smokers are affected by coronary heart disease. In this disease, the blood vessels that supply the heart are constricted, and the heart muscle does not get enough oxygen. Nicotine plays a key role here since it causes the blood vessels to narrow and increases the heart's activity.

Tobacco smoke can also be responsible for the development of angina pectoris. The symptoms of angina pectoris, literally translated as chest tightness, are seizure-like chest pain caused by a heart muscle's temporary circulatory disorder. The symptoms can also manifest themselves as a burning sensation, pain radiating from the chest region and up to the arms. The symptoms are more likely to occur in cold temperatures and after a long meal. Angina pectoris pain is closely related to coronary heart disease, as it is caused by an undersupply of oxygen to the heart muscle. In the worst case, angina pectoris can lead to a heart attack.

Smoking also increases the risk of a stroke. The toxins in cigarette smoke make the blood more viscous, and blood clots' formation is more likely. If a blood vessel in the brain is blocked, there is a lack of oxygen, and the stroke occurs.

Smoker's leg

The cause of the so-called smoker's leg lies in arteriosclerosis, i.e., hardening of the legs' blood vessels. The tar from cigarettes is deposited on the walls of the blood vessels and constricts them. The portion is no longer sufficiently supplied with blood and oxygen, and an arterial occlusive disease develops, which in the worst case, necessitates amputation.

Diseases from gums and teeth to dental decay

Smoking promotes the destruction of teeth and gums. Caries and periodontitis are a common phenomenon. If the pathogenic bacteria spread, this can lead to pneumonia, heart attacks, and strokes.

Smoke damage during pregnancy and lactation

Smoking harms the unborn child in many ways. Since 1957 there have been thousands of studies on smoking during pregnancy. Stopping smoking has various positive effects on the health and development of the child. Among other things, the probability of premature and stillbirth and sudden infant death is significantly reduced. Also, stopping smoking reduces the risk that the child is mentally and physically underdeveloped and that lung function is impaired. Overall, the blood circulation and the oxygen and nutrient supply to the embryo are vastly improved by the mother's not smoking.

Third-hand smoke - the hidden poison

When talking about smoking, passive smoking is often used, which is the smoke that people breathe in directly from the air in the room without smoking themselves. In addition to this, there is, however, an additional, so-called third-hand Smoke or "cold smoke." In the past, this hardly received any attention but has been discussed more often recently.

The cold smoke settles on different surfaces in all rooms where smoking is practiced. It also acts directly on the skin, hair, and clothing of smokers. For example, if you work at the checkout in the supermarket and go on a smoke break, you will slowly release the toxins into your environment.

An experiment[4] was conducted on third-hand smoke indoors in a German cinema where smoking was not permitted for 15 years. Researchers from Yale University and the Max Planck Institute for Chemistry, under the direction of Drew Gentner, measured the air quality inside a movie theater in Mainz for four days. As soon as they entered the cinema, the level of pollutants rose sharply. The contaminants were emitted into the room air mainly through the smokers' clothing who had smoked a cigarette before the film. The researchers could determine that the pollutant load during a film corresponds to converted ten cigarettes, which one would take up through passive smoking.

Third-hand smoke is particularly problematic in nursing professions, as patients are directly confronted with smoking caregivers' toxins. Unfortunately, the proportion of smokers in this professional environment is very high, which is very much related to the cigarette's false image as an anti-stress aid. Through smoking, the nursing staff hopes to achieve relaxation and recreation in this psychologically and physically demanding profession, which is, however, an illusion, as is well known. In any case, non-smoking can have a lot of positive effects in this area. Generally speaking, it is essential to ventilate indoor rooms as much as possible; of course, this also applies to your home.

Systematic preparation as a basis for a lasting non-smoking life

You could now stop smoking right away. It seems evident at first glance. There is nothing to stop you from quitting smoking as quickly as possible.

However, this method carries a high risk of relapse in the long run because you lack essential preparations for stopping smoking, which will help you stay permanently smoke-free.

Therefore, I have put together some preparatory measures, which have also helped me a lot. Allow yourself a total of 5 days for the preparation. Then you can do everything necessary in peace!

Continue smoking your current amount of cigarettes in the preparation phase. However, do not see this period as a final reprieve in which you "may" smoke again! During this time, the most important thing is that you analyze yourself and your smoking habits. In the long term, this will enable you to cope much better with different situations in your non-smoking everyday life. You will then not be so quickly taken by surprise by the addiction mechanisms described above.

Planning the first smoke-free day

If possible, arrange the first non-smoking day to fall on a work-free weekend or do not fix special appointments with high-stress levels on this day. In general, try to reduce all professional and private stress situations to a minimum during the first days of withdrawal.

Stress is generally a giant nicotine trap that you have to overcome. Mark the first non-smoking day in your calendar and fix this date as a reminder on your cell phone, so you will not be embarrassed to delay your smoking cessation forever.

Set up a schedule for the first smoke-free day. Write down all activities of the day and stick to it as closely as possible. Schedule activities that you enjoy doing. Of course, there is the Corona crisis, e.g., going to the cinema will not be possible at the moment. In any case, lots of exercise in the fresh air is helpful on the first day. Plan meals that you particularly enjoy eating and do as much as possible to combine them with real enjoyment and relaxation.

Look forward to your first day without cigarettes, and be proud of yourself for taking the first step towards becoming a non-smoker.

Self-analysis as a smoker

The analysis of your smoking habits is the central point in preparation for stopping smoking. This self-analysis includes two areas of your smoking life:

- The analysis of your past as a smoker

- The self-observation and analysis of your current smoking behavior

The better you know yourself and your motives for smoking, the better you will get along in the future.

The analysis of your past as a smoker

Write a short biography about your life as a smoker, describing essential stages in your smoking life so far. Find out what your original motivation was to start smoking: Were you an enthusiastic smoker from the very beginning, or did you slide into it? What was the primary function of the cigarette in your life? You must also write down why you are still smoking today, i.e., what of the previously described smoking propaganda is still affecting you. In any case, you have always had a particular fascination with smoking. Find out what smoking is supposed to give you in your life and realize that smoking is only an illusion.

Perhaps you have always been exposed to intense peer pressure and were surrounded by many smokers as a child. Maybe you are generally someone who still lets himself be talked into everything, although he has different wishes and ideas for his life? High time to gain strong self-confidence as a non-smoker and finally say no!

Did you smoke a lot from the beginning, or did you slowly increase the dose of nicotine step by step? Perhaps you tend to do things excessively? Then it is generally time to shift down a gear. Especially breathing and relaxation exercises are a great help here. More about this later.

If you have ever tried to quit but relapsed, analyze the reasons for this. You need to know the triggers, i.e., why you picked up a cigarette! Was it an extreme stress situation that caught you unprepared? Or was it a typical situation that happened again and again? Did you once again become the victim of your boss so that you "had to" reach for a cigarette due to all the stress? Or was the cigarette only too tempting to your favorite whisky with coke?

Think carefully about why you decided to stop smoking. Was it the unconditional urge to quit smoking, or did you spontaneously decide to do so more on a whim at the turn of the year? Or was it just a bit to see who could last longer? You need to develop a strong personal motivation to quit smoking. Quitting just for the benefit of another person is not enough in the long run.

Of course, it is legitimate to keep your hands off a ciga-rette, for example, because of a pregnancy, but the main thing is that you want to free yourself from tobacco smoke out of the most profound inner conviction!

Self-observation and analysis of your current smoking habits

The better you know yourself as a smoker, the more effectively you can pass through high addiction pressure situations when switching to non-smoking. Start your self-observation as a smoker today! Please observe all smoking situations during the next days of the preparation phase according to the following criteria:

Description of the respective situation

Like any smoker, you reach for a cigarette in certain situations, the place and time of day are decisive, and whether you are alone or not. The number of people around you can significantly influence whether you are stressed or not, which has a direct effect on your smoking behavior.

The function of the cigarette

The cigarette's primary function is the same for all smokers: namely the satisfaction of nicotine addiction. However, the smoker still adds individual parts. Are you, for example, primarily a stress smoker? Or should the cigarette increasingly erase the dull moments in your life?

Addiction pressure before reaching for a cigarette

Classify the addictive pressure that you feel in each situation. Use a scale from 1-5, with 5 being the highest pressure. For most smokers, the first cigarette in the morning is mainly linked to nicotine addiction, as the nicotine level has already fallen sharply again overnight.

Number of cigarettes in each situation

Furthermore, the amount of cigarettes you smoke in a particular situation is significant. There are situations in which smokers consume a whole cascade of cigarettes. For example, do you smoke a cigarette during a pleasant meeting for coffee, or do you smoke one cigarette after the other?

I smoked down half a pack in a short time when I was sitting comfortably with friends.

How does your mood change after a cigarette? How long does it take after a cigarette until you think about a new one? Maybe you don't even give the pack out of your hand after a cigarette? Do you specifically avoid certain activities to be able to smoke the next one "in time"? The more precisely you analyze your smoking habits, the more specifically you can take action against your previous behavior. You will then know which situations you need to pay particular attention to.

You can also summarize the whole thing in the form of a table, which you can find on the next page and looks like this

My smoking habits				
Situation	Function of the ciga-rette	Addiction pressure (1-5)	Number of cigarettes	Mood after the ciga-rette

This self-observations ultimate goal is to make you aware of how much nicotine manipulates you and ruins your life. After these five days, you should be glad to get out of the hostage-taking of nicotine finally.

Get misconceptions about smoking out of your head!

Long before you have reached for a cigarette for the first time, various myths about smoking have been fed into your brain. All these alleged advantages of the cigarette turn out to be false on closer inspection. It is necessary to get this nonsense out of your head. I have written down and refuted the most common misconceptions about smoking.

👎 Smoking makes slim

This myth is undoubtedly the most widespread of all. In reality, even in the long run, smoking leads to over-weight. That confirms a Viennese study[5] from the year 2014, which was published in the British Medical Journal. In this study, the health data of 986 Austrian bank em-ployees were evaluated. The scientists found out that regular smokers weigh on average 10 kilograms more and exercise less than non-smokers.

A second Finnish study[6] conducted by the Department of Public Health in Helsinki in 2009 also showed that women who smoked as teenagers started smoking in their hips in their mid-20s. Women who had smoked more than ten cigarettes a day in their teens were twice as likely to be overweight as non-smokers. Among the male participants in the study, both smokers and non-smokers built up overweight in equal measure.

👎 Smoking relaxes

From smokers, one hears again and again that they would relax with cigarettes. From the smoker's subjective point of view, this statement seems to be consistent. Whenever smokers are excited or tense, they consume a cigarette and feel more relaxed afterward.

From the outside, however, the whole thing looks different. In reality, you, as a smoker, have a continuously increased stress level due to the nicotine compulsion. This withdrawal stress is only temporarily calmed by smoking a cigarette. You always start at a higher stress level before the cigarette than a non-smoker! Through the cigarette, you will reach the maximum level that you would have automatically as a non-smoker!

Apart from that, a stressful situation will never resolve itself anyway because you are pulling toxic tobacco smoke into your lungs!

ⓓ   Smoking promotes concentration at work

This myth persists. From the smoker's perspective, this assertion seems to be accurate at first glance. Whenever the smoker becomes restless and nervous, and his thoughts slip away, he lights a cigarette and suddenly becomes focused on his work.

But as with the connection between smoking and relaxation, the situation is entirely different from concentration at second glance. Due to the constant addictive pressure of nicotine, your thoughts are always directed to the nicotine supply. In addition, the carbon monoxide supplies the brain with less oxygen, and the blood circulation is worse due to the nicotine. All in all, smoking reduces concentration.

ⓓ   Smoking a little does not harm

There is no harmless amount of cigarettes when smoking! Every cigarette contains more than 250 toxic substances, whereas tobacco smoke contains more than 70 proven carcinogenic substances!

In 2018, a study[7] on the effects of smoking concerning heart attacks and strokes was conducted and published in the British Medical Journal. It shows that smokers have an approximately 50% higher risk of heart disease from just one cigarette per day and a 30% higher risk of stroke than non-smokers.

Even if you smoke every day, your health risk after stopping smoking will be lower than that of an occasional smoker who smokes little.

In general, the image of the so-called occasional smoker is a hazardous one. Some smokers consider themselves non-smokers who only take a cigarette "for fun" one or two times. That was true for me as well, until I increasingly became a constant smoker.

👎 Light cigarettes generally cause less damage

This myth is still widespread. However, as a study[8] by Ohio State University from 2017 shows, light cigarettes, i.e., cigarettes with less tar and nicotine, have no health benefit. They even carry a higher risk of lung cancer. That's because of the additional holes in the cigarette filter, making the smoke less harsh so that the smoker automatically inhales more deeply.

👎 Stopping smoking during pregnancy damages the unborn child

This assertion is entirely absurd because tobacco smoke harms the expectant child in many ways and cannot be stopped early enough. Nicotine alone has a very toxic effect on the future child. Since 1957 there have been thousands of studies on smoking during pregnancy. Quitting smoking has various positive effects on the health and development of the child. Among other things, the probability of premature and stillbirth and sudden infant death is significantly reduced. Besides, stopping smoking reduces the risk that the child is mentally and physically underdeveloped and that lung function is impaired. The blood circulation and the embryo's oxygen and nutrient supply are also significantly improved by the mother's not smoking.

👎 **With vitamin preparations, I can protect myself as a smoker against diseases**

First, the idea does not seem to supply itself as smokers with additional vitamin preparations, not strangely, since the cigarette's poison materials reduce the reserve of micronutrients in the body. However, studies show a very counterproductive effect concerning vitamins.

A French study[9] from the year 2005 determined that the additional income of beta carotin-containing preparations, which are converted in the body to vitamin A, promotes lung cancer in smokers. By the payment of middle quantities of beta carotin-containing practices, the cancer risk increased by 43%, while with high amounts, the cancer risk even doubled.

Also, regarding vitamin E, an American study[10] from the year 2008 showed that additionally taken vitamin E preparations promote lung cancer.

☟ I've been smoking for so long anyway. There's no point in stopping!

This statement is entirely wrong because the body starts the cleaning process immediately after the last cigarette.

After only 20 minutes, a stop smoking will cause your blood pressure to normalize. In general, your organs are better supplied with blood and nutrients. Overall, your susceptibility to infections is immediately reduced, and your immune system becomes more robust.

After about 8 hours, the carbon monoxide level drops significantly, and the oxygen supply increases strongly. Already after 24 hours after stopping smoking, the risk of heart attack begins to decrease gradually. Within a year, you have only half the risk of coronary heart disease.

In addition, coughing and sputum gradually diminish over the next few months, after the lungs' self-purification may have temporarily increased them. Your arteries become increasingly elastic over the next few months. Overall, you can significantly improve your health within a year.

Always keep the following in mind:

As a non-smoker, you do not renounce a precious life with cigarettes, but as a smoker, you lose a free and happy life without cigarettes!

The supposed pleasure of smoking is, in reality, nothing more than the satisfaction of nicotine addiction, which systematically makes you poison yourself. The cigarette is nothing more than a radioactive, chemical poison stick!

The nicotine can make you believe what it wants, smoking will only harm you in the long run, but as a non-smoker, you have numerous advantages, as you will see in a moment!

Anchoring the advantages of not smoking in the mind

In this section, I would like to show you now that your life as a non-smoker will be better in every respect, no matter how long you have been a smoker! You will enjoy these benefits every day, and the longer you keep your hands off cigarettes, the more you will realize how absurd smoking has been.

In the following, I have written down the various advantages that you should keep in mind:

✓ You will wake up fresher and more relaxed right at the beginning of the day because your circulation and oxygen supply are better.

✓ Your energy level will be higher throughout the day due to the increased oxygen and blood circulation.

- ✓ When you wake up, you no longer smell as if you had slept in an ashtray.

- ✓ You no longer have the feeling of having eaten out of an ashtray in the morning.

- ✓ In the morning, you will no longer have red and burning eyes.

- ✓ Your lungs finally begin to cleanse themselves as your bronchi are no longer polluted with toxic tobacco smoke.

- ✓ You will soon have no more headaches from smoking, as the blood circulation in your head, and the oxygen supply are continually improving.

- ✓ Your hands are not always unpleasantly cold because the blood circulation in your hands improves.

- ✓ Your breakfast smells and tastes right again. As a smoker, you have increasingly dulled your senses.

- ✓ Your gums and teeth begin to regenerate, gum bleeding, and tooth destruction is stopped.

- ✓ Your home is no longer a smoking cave. The poisonous smoke can no longer accumulate on all surfaces every day.

✓ There are no more smelly, smoky clothes hanging in your apartment, which emits toxic cold smoke.

✓ Your car is no longer a moving smoking chamber. It does not stink all the time, and your seats are no longer full of toxic, cold smoke.

✓ They no longer appear as a walking ashtray at the workplace or the customer's premises.

✓ Long meetings or meetings with customers are much more relaxed because the addiction pressure is gone.

✓ Under time pressure, you have more room to maneuver for important work without cigarette breaks.

✓ You won't come back to your workplace in an ash cloud after every break in your work.

✓ During the break, you can relax and eat something useful instead of satisfying your nicotine addiction in the smoking area.

✓ As a non-smoker, you can work much more concentrated and calmer because the craving for nicotine does not always distract your thoughts.

✓ After a hard day's work, you won't come back to a stinking, smoky apartment where you will be fogged in again.

- ✓ You can go to any smoke-free restaurant and enjoy the food again.

- ✓ The stay in smoke-free rooms will be relaxed again, even if the film has no break despite its excess length.

- ✓ A walk in the forest becomes a wellness and sensory experience again because you can smell adequately too.

- ✓ You'll never have to go out to smoke at a party again.

- ✓ You gain a lot of disease-free lifetime through the health effects of not smoking. On average, smokers are more often ill than non-smokers.

- ✓ With each saved cigarette, you gain about 3-4 minutes of your daily lifetime, which you can use for other useful things.

- ✓ If you save ten cigarettes a day, you gain an average of 9.4 years of life expectancy as a man and 7.3 years as a woman.

- ✓ You travel relaxed again. Long bus journeys no longer become compulsive, waiting for the next rest stop to provide nicotine replenishment.

- ✓ You can also sit back and relax during long train rides or flights, although flying is, of course, currently not possible in the Corona crisis.

✓ You can go sightseeing on vacation without being confronted continuously with smoking bans.

✓ You can enjoy the fresh breeze by the sea without inhaling toxic tobacco smoke.

✓ You don't get out of breath immediately when you want to go for a little hike.

✓ In everyday life, the stairs lose their horror when, for example, the elevator of the residential complex is down again.

✓ For example, you save 5 euros per cigarette pack in Austria and 6 euros in Germany. If you put 5 Euro on your side every day, you will save 1800 Euro per year. You can save something for later financial difficulties, especially now in the crisis

✓ You can afford small rewards every day instead of smoking cigarettes out the window.

✓ You will have health benefits from not smoking right from the start. After only 20 minutes, your blood pressure normalizes, and your circulation stabilizes.

✓ Your immune system will improve immediately because the negative effect of smoking on white blood cells is eliminated. The probability of pneumonia is also reduced when you stop smoking.

- ✓ As current studies on the coronavirus, including those from China, show, smokers are much more likely to suffer a severe course of the infectious disease. As I said, now is absolutely the right time to stop smoking!

- ✓ All organs are better supplied with oxygen, and the risk of cancer is significantly reduced.

- ✓ Your basic physical condition improves due to improved blood circulation and oxygen supply.

- ✓ In 48 hours, the carbon monoxide will have almost completely disappeared from your body, and you will be able to breathe more air again.

- ✓ Your risk of heart attack and stroke will decrease after just 24 hours.

- ✓ Your skin is much better supplied with oxygen and nutrients and looks healthier.

- ✓ Their sexual health improves dramatically; infertility and potency problems are much more common among smokers.

- ✓ You gain self-confidence because you control your life again, and your overall mental health improves.

Inform my environment

Be sure to tell your environment that you want to become a non-smoker, including your professional colleagues. On the one hand, you can get support for your project; on the other hand, you allow your environment to adjust. By making your smoking cessation public, you create positive pressure from outside, which helps you implement your plans.

Set up a smoke stop hotline with your best friends, where your helpers are always available, especially if you are struggling with intense withdrawal symptoms.

Ask your friends to be considerate of you and not to smoke in front of you. As mentioned in the previous chapter, smoking role models have a powerful influence on others. Tell your smoking friends that you don't want to go to smoking establishments under any circumstances and that parties with alcohol and cigarettes are taboo for the time being.

Contacts to other ex-smokers, with whom they can also exchange information about the smoking stop, are also very positive. Through the community feeling, you are strengthened in your way as a non-smoker. This is precisely the opposite model to your previous life as a smoker, in which you were motivated to smoke by a community.

Smoking the very last cigarette

On the 5th day of your preparation phase, the time has come: for the very last time in your life, you will consume this poisonous rod called a cigarette and then finally be free.

If possible, smoke your very last cigarette in the evening before going to bed so that you are nicotine-free the next morning. Create a quiet environment at home and concentrate on that crucial moment.

Now make yourself fully aware of what smoking does to your body and psyche, taste and smell the tobacco smoke consciously for the next few minutes:

Light the glow stick and pull on it. Watch how the poisonous smoke flows through your mouth, throat, and deep down into your lungs, spreads, and irritates your airways. Remember how toxic this smoke is and what it does to you every time you breathe it.

Feel the smoke on your tongue and taste it. Smack it a few times correctly and take this disgusting taste of poisonous and stinking ashes! You will soon realize how absurd the claim that smoking tastes good is!

Pay attention to the smoking cigarette and remember how toxic the tobacco smoke you are currently inhaling is. Think again of all the radioactive and chemical substances that are dispersed in the air at that moment.

Remember that the nicotine is now constricting your blood vessels and your veins are full of the poison. With every puff of a cigarette, you spread this poison through-out your body!

However, the nicotine is currently docking on the nico-tine receptors in your head, trying to distract you from your self-intoxication. Again, it plays its manipulative game with dopamine and endorphins and pretends to bring you fun and happiness. Ignore this illusion and think now about all the benefits you will enjoy after this very last cigarette!

Now draw the last toxic residue into the body until only the filter is left and make yourself aware once and for all, how disgusting smoking is. And then squeeze out that awful stuff for the last time!

Congratulations! You have finally drawn the line! Open the window wide and breathe deeply. You have com-pleted your 5-day preparation phase, and your new life as a non-smoker has begun! Enter the end of your smok-ing life with a smiley face in the calendar right now. In 24 hours, you can draw the next smiley!

The best thing to do now is take an extensive shower and wash the ashes off your body. Relax and look forward to your first smoke-free day! Now you can make your home smoke-free.

Finally, create a smoke-free environment

Do the following in your new non-smoking life:

Collect the whole cigarette stocks at home, including any leftover cigarettes in the car, and throw them into the nearest dustbin in front of the house. Also, remove all smoking utensils such as ashtrays and lighters. Be aware, these items are closely linked to your addiction memory and can put you back on the wrong track!

Then wash all curtains, upholstery, and blankets over the next few days. Wipe everything in your apartment, including all floors. This will reduce the cold smoke that has accumulated on the surfaces. It has also been collected on your clothes and is slowly spreading throughout your home. Ventilate regularly to get rid of the toxic smoke particles little by little.

The next chapter will now focus on the strategies you can establish as a non-smoker from day one.

Success strategies from the first day as a non-smoker

The following strategies have made me a successful non-smoker until today. Please implement them consistently step by step. The most important thing now is that you approach the matter with positive thoughts and relax as best you can.

Successfully to the durable non-smoker in 24 - hours - steps

At my "best times" as a smoker, I could not imagine a day without tobacco smoke. My life was literally in a fog.

Today the whole thing looks completely different. I can't even imagine pulling a cigarette today, so smoking disgusts me. There is no room for it in my head anymore, and I have something better to do every second than poisoning myself with cigarettes

But to get there in the long run, you first have to proceed in small steps. The key to success is to think in 24-hour steps. Concentrate on your first day as a non-smoker. Take the plan you created in the preparation phase and implement it step by step. Once you have done that, you can proudly pat yourself on the back. Repeat this success repeatedly until it has become entirely normal to get up in the morning and not smoke all day. Tell yourself inwardly every time you wake up:

TODAY I AM NON-SMOKER AND TOMORROW I WILL BE THE SAME!

This 24-hour routine will help you, especially if you have a mental sag in the first weeks. Make yourself aware that you can achieve further success in a few hours at a time and follow through with your 24-hour program consistently. With each day, you store new non-smoking experiences in your brain, and after a few weeks, these will be firmly anchored in your long-term memory.

Avoid dicey places and situations from the outset

Especially in the beginning, you can save yourself a lot of stress if you avoid certain places and situations with foresight. I have written down the most important ones below.

Currently, in the corona crisis, the first two points inevitably fall away, depending on how intense the relaxation in your place of residence is. But after the crisis, you must avoid all subsequent situations in the long run systematically.

- Smoking cafés and smoking bars

Here you are doubly stressed, on the one hand, by smoking role models and, on the other hand, by breathing in passive smoke. Do not visit such places, especially in the first months.

General smoking bans help a lot here. For example, a public smoking ban in restaurants and bars has been in force in Austria since November 1st, 2019. One can only hope that corresponding regulations will be enforced in other EU countries and worldwide.

- Parties without smoker control

Straight house parties without smoke restriction are particularly unfavorable. Here you have the same scenario as in smoking establishments, with usually much more alcohol flowing. If you plan to have a party later in the future, I recommend the strict rule that smokers are only allowed to smoke outside.

- Smoking area at the workplace

As mentioned earlier, the smoking area is the worst possible place to stop smoking. It is better to get something delicious to eat during your break and get moving. Or go to the non-smoking area of your company. There you can talk to non-smokers just as well.

- Tobacco Shops

Your addiction memory will be activated there as well. Every smoker has the memory of having bought cigarettes in a tobacconist's shop. Besides, the particular advertising design of the tobacconist's is a big problem: On the one hand, you see all cigarette brands on the presentation plate in front of you. On the other hand, advertising posters hang in front of you, and lighters and ashtrays are everywhere. Also, promoters sometimes advertise cigarettes directly on site. So it's best to buy your newspapers or recharging slips for your cell phone at the supermarket or cell phone store.

Introducing new non-smoking habits and getting rid of old smoking habits

From the first day as a non-smoker, get your body moving instead of sitting around with a cigarette. On the one hand, exercise is optimal to reduce stress as the body secretes happiness hormones. On the other hand, your circulation gets going, and you can get more oxygen. Especially the oxygen intake has suffered all the time due to smoking. Extended walks are beneficial.

Especially in the morning, replace the first cigarette after waking up with a walk in the fresh air! Fill your stressed lungs with plenty of oxygen right at the beginning of the day; your heart and circulation will thank you! You can also get something fresh from the bakery. Then you will have taken a few steps right away.

Get moving even during work breaks. Even a short up and down of the stairs will get your circulation going. Even in the evening after work, take a walk and let the day pass in peace.

Of course, it would be ideal to find a hobby where you can move around a lot. Maybe you used to pursue a hobby you gave up because of smoking, such as swimming or table tennis. You can also go jogging once or twice a week, but I strongly advise you to have a thorough medical examination or seek ongoing advice.

Nutrient-rich food instead of tobacco smoke

Especially important when switching from smoking to non-smoking is the diet. Supply yourself now with many vitamins and nutrients so that you can support your body massively in regeneration.

If you are a passionate coffee drinker and have always smoked a cigarette, drink the coffee first, and replace the cigarette with dental chewing gum with xylitol.

If you're not that enthusiastic about coffee anyway, you can replace it with a cup of your favorite tea. After dinner, you can also enjoy a cup of tea.

I have put together a list of foods that systematically promote your physical and psychological well-being. Please pay attention to any allergies you may have and, if in doubt, omit the respective food. In general, however, everything should be very well tolerated.

- Red onions

Contain sulfides and the plant dye quercetin. Quercetin is proven to be anti-cancer and has a strong anti-inflammatory effect. Of all vegetables, onions have the highest concentration of the flavonoid quercetin, especially in the outer skin.

- Cabbage vegetables

Especially red cabbage has a very positive influence on health through its mustard oils and plant dyes. These ingredients open the blood vessels, have an anti-inflammatory effect, and boost the immune system.

- Coconut and coconut water

The flesh of the coconut contains many minerals and antioxidants. However, do not overeat the coconut's meat, as it is very high in calories. The lauric acid it contains is antimicrobial, has an anti-inflammatory effect, and cleanse the body. Coconut water also has a lot of potassium for stable blood pressure and is a low-calorie alternative to the flesh.

- Carrots

This vegetable is known to contain a lot of vitamin A for the skin and mucous membranes and a lot of fiber. These help you to excrete cholesterol and lower blood lipids.

- Naturally, cloudy apple juice

Mainly, cloudy apple juice contains many minerals, vitamins, and other health-promoting substances such as polyphenols. These plant substances prevent heart disease and intestinal cancer. Besides, apple juice contains so-called pectins, which support lung function.

- Sea buckthorn juice

Like the red onion, sea buckthorn contains many highly effective plant substance quercetins, vitamin C and A for a robust immune system. Since sea buckthorn tastes very tart, I recommend drinking it together with a sweet fruit juice, e.g., apple juice.

- Mineral water with hydrogen carbonate

Drinking lots of mineral water supports circulation and dilutes the blood. Hydrogen carbonate, also called baking soda, has an anti-inflammatory and immune-soothing effect.

- Potatoes

contain many vitamin C, are very good for the bronchial tubes, protect the intestines, and promote digestion. Potatoes provide easily digestible carbohydrates without making you fat.

- Bananas

contain antioxidants like catechins. They are high in potassium, thus regulating blood pressure and protecting the heart. Bananas are also an excellent source of carbohydrates and will keep you full.

- Kale

It provides many minerals, especially calcium, and vitamins, such as vitamin C or K. It contains a lot of antioxidants and minerals. Kale improves the flow properties of the blood and is anti-inflammatory.

- Salmon

Eat wild salmon if possible. It contains Omega 3 fatty acids, vitamins D and E, and essential amino acids. Salmon is very anti-inflammatory and provides perfect protein. Salmon is very healthy, especially for the lungs.

- Linseed oil

Linseed oil is an excellent source of omega-three fatty acids, which provides far more omega-three fatty acids than fish. Linseed oil promotes a healthy cholesterol household and lowers blood pressure. The polyphenols work anti-oxidatively, and the plant connections work cancer restraining.

- Eggs (especially the yolk)

Eggs contain many essential nutrients, e.g., vitamin D or vitamin A. They have optimally digestible proteins and promote good cholesterol.

Besides, I can recommend ivy products for the bronchial tubes if you have a cold or cough. Especially as a former smoker, you generally have a damaged bronchial tube. Ivy has a very positive effect on your strained mucous membranes and opens your pulmonary alveoli. Healing salt tablets like Emser Salz (salt) is also very soothing for the mucous membranes.

Addiction attacks and what you can do about them

The addiction attacks, the so-called cravings, are the most challenging moments during withdrawal. In these situations, your thoughts only revolve around cigarettes. However, these Cravings last only 2 minutes on average. With the right antidotes, which I will show you in a moment, you can consistently ward them off. In principle, breathing exercises and movement exercises are the most effective. But there are also other remedies that you can use successfully.

Essential in a psychological addiction attack is not to go into panic mode. Don't try to suppress the addictive thoughts doggedly; you will only increase the stress!

It is about steering your thoughts entirely away from smoking, concentrating on a different action, and relaxing overall. I can recommend the following tools to help you get through these situations successfully:

Breathing exercises

There are two simple but very effective exercises. These help you to regain peace and balance.

Exercise 1:

This exercise is especially useful when you are on the road. Stand upright and take 20 slow deep breaths in and out. Breathe through your nose. Concentrate on how your lungs and abdomen are deeply filled with oxygen. Imagine that you systematically breathe the thoughts of smoking out of your body. It is best to do this exercise in front of an open window if you are at home.

Exercise 2:

When you are at home, lie down on a mat on the floor and breathe in and out deeply 20 times. Let your body sink, relaxed. Imagine your body being pulled apart like a rubber band. Pay close attention to how your lungs are filled with oxygen and imagine how you exhale smoking thoughts.

Movement during addiction attacks

As I said, movement, in general, plays a prominent role in withdrawal. Especially if you are sitting in the office at work and are struck by an addiction attack, take a break and go out into the fresh air if possible. Do breathing exercises one and relax. If you are at home in such a situation, go outside if possible, weather permitting. If not, you can go back to the breathing exercises.

Friends - Hotline

It helps you a lot if you are frequently in contact with friends from your environment. Especially now in the corona crisis, friends are doubly valuable. Of course, it is essential that this friend is very reliable and that he or she is always available. Describe your current situation to your conversation partner so that he or she can respond to you as well as possible. The conversation alone makes time pass, and the addiction attack will soon be over.

Activities in which you cannot smoke.

- put under the shower for a few minutes
- turn around with the wheel (possibly limited possible)
- go jogging, if you have the medical permission
- go swimming (currently not possible)
- Drink a glass of water or fruit juice

Drinking is especially vital in withdrawal. On the one hand, it helps you physically, as it is good for the circulation, dilutes the blood, and helps the body flush out the toxic substances.

On the other hand, drinking can also help you get over a mental addiction attack. Whenever the addiction besieges you, pour yourself a glass of water or fruit juice as calmly as possible and drink it down slowly. Breathe as calmly and relaxed as possible. Soon the haunting will be over.

Dental care chewing gums with xylitol

These gums can be chewed throughout the day and can also be used when you are not under the influence of addiction. Dental care chewing gums have a double positive effect: On the one hand, you can distract your smoking thoughts by chewing. On the other hand, you clean your teeth, which have been badly affected by smoking. You can get these chewing gums mainly in health food stores or online mail order.

Chewing toothpicks

If you do not have a dental chewing gum at hand, you can also use a toothpick. Chew on it evenly during an addiction attack. This will help you get over the time of the attack. However, the toothpick is not suitable for permanent use. Never chew on a toothpick for more than 30 minutes a day, as this can cause tension and pain in the jaw.

In everyday life, try to breathe calmly and deeply and spare your nerves. Try to relax more often. The higher your chances will be to get rid of cigarettes finally.

Every time you say no to a cigarette, you deepen your non-smoking memory and train your non-smoking routines. If an addiction attack should strike you, you now have the necessary remedies at hand.

Keep a written record of your non-smoking life

From the first non-smoking day on, make a short non-smoking protocol by recording the previous day's experiences. Write down the most critical stages of the day in rough outlines. Describe when you felt good and where you experienced problems or possibly a strong addiction attack. Also, write down which strategies worked best for you.

Think about what you can improve in the future. For example, you could get up even earlier the next day gain a little more time for breakfast in the morning. That way, you will have less stress.

In the evening, you can review the day again by writing down your non-smoking experiences. On the one hand, this is a confirmation of your day's success, and on the other hand, it is comparable to a captain's logbook, which you can use to orientate yourself again and again.

The successes that you record every day will give you self-confidence and make you proud. So it easier for you to motivate yourself anew every time, even when you are mentally down.

It is also beneficial to look back in the records and see how the whole thing has developed over days and weeks.

Set up a non-smoker account

There will be a lot of money to be made once you stop smoking. Meanwhile, a pack of cigarettes costs about 6 dollars in America. You pay more for two packs of cigarettes a day than you would for one movie, and that every day of the month.

You can either put this money aside or, in any case, invest it better than in cigarettes. It is best to deposit the money that has so far dissolved into tobacco smoke into a separate non-smoker account. Set up a monthly standing order on this account. On average, you can put away 5 euros per day. As already mentioned in the previous chapter on the advantages of not smoking, you will have over 150 euros per month and 1800 euros per year! In the current crisis, every euro is twice as valuable.

Use this money to make small rewards for yourself now and then and be proud that you have made the right decision for your life.

Preventing a shift in addiction

Some new ex-smokers try to compensate for the "missing" nicotine kick with another addiction. In the back of your mind, there is still the idea that you need something to cope with problems or to have fun.

In the case of an addiction shift, you suddenly carry out activities that you have previously done to a usual extent excessively. For example, you may become a workaholic, become obsessed with cleaning, develop an eating addiction, or resort to alcohol. As a smoker, you have to be careful with alcohol and food, as these things have been strongly linked to your smoking behavior.

Alcohol addiction

Alcohol and cigarettes go together very well in the wrong way. Both drugs act on the same nerve cells and reinforce each other. Besides, nicotine makes you less tired from drinking alcohol, so smokers will unconsciously drink more alcohol.

You have probably also already made the experience that you automatically smoked more when consuming alcohol and that you "tasted" the cigarettes with alcohol better. If you skip cigarettes in the future, you may get the feeling that you are "missing" something and suddenly drink more alcohol. The subconscious mind and your addiction memory trigger this behavior.

Especially at the beginning of your non-smoking life, you must, therefore, be careful not to consume more alcoholic beverages. It is best to drink as little or no alcohol as possible in the beginning and then reduce your alcohol consumption in the long term. It makes no sense to celebrate your smokelessness with more alcohol in the future.

If you replace cigarettes with dental chewing gum after a beer, you create a suitable cigarette alternative.

Eating addiction, especially sweets

Many non-smokers initially tend to consume more sugary foods. Some of them eat several packs of jelly babies in a row. This can be explained by the fact that there are some striking parallels between eating and cigarette smoking, especially when it comes to sweets:

- You open a package for sweets and cigarettes and put the contents directly into your mouth with your hand.

- Sugar works as fast as nicotine.

- In both cases, one satisfies a "hunger," whereby the feeling of satiety does not last long.

- In principle, both are available everywhere very quickly.

Some ex-smokers report that after stopping smoking, they increase or risk increasing. Eat, therefore, as previously mentioned, in the future, somewhat smaller meals and more vegetables and fruit. Although you do not have to do without sugar altogether, you should not eat large quantities of sugar at once.

There is a simple solution to gaining weight: if you get more exercise, your calorie consumption will increase. Think of stairs as fitness equipment. Leave your car at home more often, and do your shopping on foot if possible.

How to master existential crises without relapse

As mentioned at the beginning, we are currently in a particular crisis that affects many areas of our lives. Although we naturally hope that we will survive this crisis and possible, it can lead to various existential crises for us, which are connected with a high-stress factor. These crises include:

- Job loss

- Divorce

- Death/accident of a close relative

- Diagnosis of a disease (currently of course also Covid 19)

In all these incidents, a shock situation can bring you very close to the threshold of a relapse. A veritable flood of stress is created, which can activate your addiction memory in a flash. The categories of stress management and smoking are stored together in this memory, which makes such situations particularly challenging. The cigarette will once again appear as a false helper, but no matter how much tobacco smoke you draw into your lungs, it will not help you at all!

It is best to resort to breathing exercises and exercise in the fresh air to avoid a relapse. Of course, emotional support from family, friends, and psychologists is especially crucial in these situations. Call your friends on your hotline as often as possible. You must always remember that smoking a cigarette will not help you solve your problems!

Try to get back on track as soon as possible and draw up a contingency plan. Don't let yourself down and focus your thoughts on positive memories and thoughts to relieve yourself mentally. Despite everything, counter the current crisis successfully as a non-smoker and systematically rewind your non-smoking routines as usual.

As soon as you have survived this state of emergency, you will emerge from the crisis with doubly strengthened self-confidence and overcome everyday situations even more naturally.

Hands off all nicotine products!

The image of smoking is increasingly on the defensive, especially in the western world. In return, more and more so-called smoke alternatives or nicotine replacement products are being advertised, which are sold to consumers as a harmless alternative to smoking. Mainly the e-cigarette is thereby at present in focus.

You probably have already thought about switching to these alternatives. It sounds temptingly simple to switch to another "luxury food" that is supposedly a healthy alternative.

However, the following problem exists: Every nicotine product brings you back into the nicotine cycle and puts you in danger of sooner or later returning to smoking! Let us take a closer look at the most common nicotine products:

E-cigarettes: Steaming with nicotine

The e-cigarette is repeatedly touted as a healthier alternative to cigarette smoking, as no tobacco is inhaled, and instead of smoke, steam is emitted from the e-cigarette. How harmful e-cigarettes are precise, cannot be determined due to missing long-term studies yet strictly; however, the e-cigarette is by no means harmless. In October 2019, cases of lung diseases in America became public, which were called in connection with the smoking of e-cigarettes[11][12]. In the USA, dozens of people died, and many others were poisoned. E-cigarettes may also contain carcinogenic substances such as benzene or formaldehyde. [13]San Francisco has meanwhile banned the manufacture and sale of e-cigarettes.

Nevertheless, the e-cigarette enjoys growing popularity worldwide, especially the so-called Juul is popular with young people. Due to its shape, this cigarette is strongly reminiscent of a USB stick and contains exceptionally high nicotine levels in the USA.

In the EU, manufacturers had to reduce the nicotine content significantly to obtain approval. Due to various additives, this e-cigarette appears unusually mild and is, therefore, incredibly tempting for beginners.

Also, the e-cigarette could serve as a gateway drug for young people to start smoking later, as the German Society for Pneumology (DGP) warned in a position paper[14] 2015.

Shisha smoking - the allegedly healthier smoking alternative

Shisha or water pipe smoking is considered by many to be a healthier way to smoke. This thesis's main argument is that the water filters out the smoke toxins in the water pipe. But this assertion is entirely absurd. The water in the shisha does not filter out the toxins but only cools the smoke, which allows the consumer to draw all the toxins even deeper into the lungs. Besides, the shisha does not have a filter like a cigarette.

The hookah tobacco does not burn but carbonizes at low temperatures, creating toxins such as acetaldehyde, acrolein, or benzene.

Tar is also produced when smoking shisha, and this is due to the smoldering of the coal. Shisha smoking creates a large amount of carbon monoxide, which spreads in the immediate vicinity. As a result, oxygen uptake becomes more difficult, which can be very problematic, especially in the long term. As one can infer from various media reports, poisoning symptoms and emergencies in Shisha-bars occur repeatedly[1516].

Many Shisha smokers trivialize the water pipe by saying that they only smoke once a month anyway. However, shisha smoking immediately reactivates the addictive memory and brings you back into the nicotine cycle into it. The shisha is often the first step into cigarette smoking, especially for young people.

Smoke hemp (cannabis)

Hemp is currently experiencing a real boom internationally. The smoking of hemp, also called cannabis, has been legalized in more and more countries worldwide in the last years. The main active ingredients of the hemp plant are THC and CBD. While THC's consumption is still illegal or highly regulated in most states, the non-psychotic CBD oil is now more and more often offered in its stores.

Smoking cannabis is often described as a harmless alternative to cigarette smoking, quasi as "medicine." However, there are many arguments against this.

On the one hand, tobacco is added to the cannabis joint, which immediately brings us back to nicotine. Here the nicotine addiction is reactivated, just like with shisha smoking.

Studies show [17] that regular cannabis smoking significantly increases testicular cancer risk and makes [18]lung cancer more likely. Smoking a joint is as devastating as smoking 20 cigarettes.

Nicotine substitutes

There are different offerers of nicotine substitutes for some years, which want to wean smokers by low-dose nicotine gifts step by step.

This method's idea is that the ex-smoker is still given nicotine, but in shallow doses and comparison to the cigarette, with a very long time delay. The amount of nicotine is then gradually reduced, and after a few weeks, it is completely stopped. The nicotine is made available to the consumer in chewing gums, sprays, patches, or inhalation devices.

At first glance, this method seems to make sense. These smoking cessation products are free of the toxins that tobacco smoke brings with it. Of course, the nicotine kick, which can quickly lead to addiction when smoking, is almost eliminated.

Despite all this, the fact remains that you are taking precisely the substance that made you dependent on smoking. Subconsciously, the following is established in your head: I need nicotine to get rid of cigarettes! You are therefore embarking on a dubious path that leads back into the nicotine swamp for many smokers.

Stay away from all of these products and enjoy your life without nicotine instead! You will see, there is nothing better for an ex-smoker than to be free of nicotine!

Watch out! Arrogance comes before the nicotine relapse!

At the end of the book, I would like to warn you once again to be careful not to become careless towards cigarettes in the future! The longer you will be smoke-free, the more dangerous will be the thought that nothing can happen to you now anyway and that a cigarette will not make you addicted again. The way out of the nicotine swamp is then already some time behind you, and smoking no longer seems to be a threat to you, according to the motto: "What could happen if I smoke one now?

Remember, those remnants of your addiction memory are still slumbering in your head! Even from your environment can come sayings like: "It's been ages since you stopped smoking, you can try one!

Theoretically, the addiction trap lurks in the most diverse emotional situations. Whether you're exultant or saddened to death, bored or angry, the craving for a cigarette can always reappear somewhere. Don't forget one thing: You can't take time out from not smoking. A puff on a cigarette ends your non-smoking life!

Therefore there is only one way as a non-smoker: Do not play with fire and do not become careless in any case! Become aware of all the advantages you have as a non-smoker and enjoy every smoke-free day!

Concluding remarks

I hope I could motivate you fully to stop smoking with this book and give you a clear direction for your future non-smoking life! If you get stuck on your way, you can always grab this book. In any case, always concentrate on the next 24-hours. Be proud of yourself as soon as you have taken your hands off your cigarette again around the clock!

You can also support me by writing a short review of my book on Amazon. On the one hand, you can tell me how you are doing as a non-smoker and, on the other hand, how you liked the book in general. My readers' criticism is essential to me, and I am happy to incorporate wishes and suggestions into future books!

To rate my book, please do the following: Go to the Amazon page and enter the search term of my book: "I do not smoke! My head is free of nicotine!". Tap on the title of my book there. Then scroll down on my book page where the following is written:

Review this product

Share your thoughts with other customers

Write a customer review

I look forward to your numerous feedback and thank you in advance for your interest and support!

All the best and above all, a long non-smoking life!

Markus K. Hoffmann

Appendix

Imprint and disclaimer

© Author Markus K. Hoffmann

1st edition 2020

All rights reserved

Reprinting, even in part, is prohibited

No part of this work may be reproduced, duplicated, or distributed in any form without the author's written permission.

Contact us: Markus Kurzemann Wagramerstrasse 95/1/7, 1220 Vienna

Cover design: Markus K. Hoffmann using the Adobe Stock Image with the No.166598222

Disclaimer

List of sources

---

[1] National Cancer Institute. The Role of the Media in Promoting and Reducing Tobacco Use. Tobacco Control Monograph No. 19. Bethesda, MD: U.S. Department of Health and Human Services, National Institutes of Health, National Cancer Institute. NIH Pub. No. 07-6242, June 2008.

[2] Maria L. Loureiro, Anna Sanz-de-Galdeano, Daniela Vuri. Smoking Habits: Like Father, Like Son, Like Mother, Like Daughter?*. Oxford Bulletin of Economics and Statistics, 2010; 72 (6): 717 DOI: 10.1111/j.1468-0084.2010.00603.x

[3] German Cancer Research Center (Ed.): Tobacco smoke - a poisonous mixture Heidelberg, 2008

[4] Roger Sheu, Christof Stönner, Jenna C. Ditto, Thomas Klüpfel, Jonathan Williams, Drew R. Gentner Human transport of thirdhand tobacco smoke: A prominent source of hazardous air pollutants into indoor nonsmoking environments, Science Advances 04 Mar 2020: Vol. 6, no. 10, eaay4109DOI: 10.1126/sciadv.aay4109

[5] de Oliveira Fontes Gasperin L, Neuberger M, Tichy A, et alCross-sectional association between cigarette smoking and abdominal obesity among Austrian bank employeesBMJOpen 2014;4:e004899. doi: 10.1136/bmjopen-2014-004899

[6] Saarni Se, Pietiläinen K, Kantonen S, Rissanen A, Kaprio J. Association of smoking in adolescence with abdominal obesity in adulthood: a follow-up study of 5 birth cohorts of Finnish twins. Am J Public Health. 2009 Feb;99(2):348-54.

[7] Ilan Hackshaw, Joan K Morris, Sadie Boniface, Jin-Ling Tang, Dušan Milenković. Low cigarette consumption and risk of coronary heart disease and stroke: meta-analysis of 141 cohort studies in 55 study reports
BMJ 2018;360:j5855doi: https://doi.org/10.1136/bmj.j5855 (Published 24 January 2018)

[8] Min-Ae Song, Neal L Benowitz, Micah Berman, Theodore M Brasky, K Michael Cummings, Dorothy K Hatsukami, Catalin Marian, Richard O'Connor, Vaughan W Rees, Casper WoroszyloNCI: Journal of the National Cancer Institute, Volume 109, Issue12, December 2017, djx075, https://doi.org/10.1093/jnci/djx075

[9] Mathilde Touvier, Emmanuelle Kesse, Françoise Clavel-Chapelon, Marie-Christine Boutron-Ruault Dual Association of β-Carotene With Risk of Tobacco-Related Cancers in a Cohort of French Women JNCI: Journal of the National Cancer Institute, Volume 97, Issue 18, 21 September 2005, Pages 1338-1344

[10] Christopher G. Slatore, Alyson J. Littman, David H. Au, Jessie A. Satia, and Emily White Long-Term Use of Supplemental Multivitamins, Vitamin C, Vitamin E, and Folate Does Not Reduce the Risk of Lung Cancer https://doi.org/10.1164/rccm.200709-1398OC

[11] t.online.de 18.10.2019.Number of deaths caused by e-cigarettes in the USA continues to rise. https://www.t-online.de/gesundheit/gesund-leben/id_86641478/e-zigaretten-zahl-der-toten-durch-lungenschaeden-in-den-usa-steigt-weiter-.html

[12] derstandard.at.25 October 2019.number of deaths from e-cigarettes in the USA increased to 34. https://www.derstand-ard.at/story/2000110313379/zahl-der-toten-durch-e-zigaretten-in-den-usa-auf

[13]German Cancer Research Center (Ed.) Tobacco Heaters. Facts about smoking, Heidelberg, 2018

[14] Nowak D et al. position paper of the German Society for Pneumology and Respiratory Medicine... Pneumology 2015; 69: 131-134

[15] kurier.at.1.04.2019.CO poisoning in shisha bar: Young people in hospital. https://kurier.at/chronik/wien/kohlenmonoxid-vergiftung-in-shisha-bar-vier-junge-menschen-im-spital/400452865

[16] rp-online.de.7.02.2019.Düsseldorf increases controls in shisha bars. https://rp-online.de/nrw/staedte/duesseldorf/immer-mehr-kohlenmonoxid-vergiftungen-in-duesseldorf-mehr-kontrollen-in-shisa-bars_aid-36604349

[17] standard.at. 9.02.2009.Cannabis promotes testicular cancer Long-term use doubles the risk of the aggressive tumor form. https://www.derstandard.at/story/1233587035229/us-studie-cannabis-foerdert-hodenkrebs

[18] lung physicians in the net.de. 07.04.2008. Cannabis more carcinogenic than tobacco. https://www.lunge-naerzte-im-netz.de/news-archiv/meldung/article/cannabis-krebs-erregender-als-tabak/

www.ingramcontent.com/pod-product-compliance
Lightning Source LLC
Chambersburg PA
CBHW061509250726

48657CB00005B/1761